The #AskDrA Book

Vol 2

Dr. Guillermo Alvarez

Rob Anspach

The #AskDrA Book

Vol 2

Easy & Practical Answers
To Enjoying Life
As A New "Sleever".

*Based On Episodes 27-52 Of The #AskDrA Show.

The #AskDrA Book - Vol 2

Published by: Anspach Media
P.O. Box 2
Conestoga PA 17516 USA

ISBN 10: 0-9894663-4-5

ISBN 13: 978-0-9894663-4-9

While they have made every effort to verify the information provided in this publication, neither the author(s) nor the publisher assumes any responsibility for errors in, omissions from or different interpretation of the subject matter.

The information herein may be subject to varying laws and practices in different areas, states and countries. The reader assumes all responsibility for use of the information.

** *Disclaimer: Individual results may vary. The statements in this book and on our website and all affiliates have not been evaluated by the FDA. Products mentioned herein are not intended to diagnose, treat, cure or prevent any disease and do not replace medical advice. Advice on treatment or care of an individual patient should be obtained through consultation with a physician or trained health care practitioner who has examined that patient or is familiar with that patient's medical history.*

Dedicated

To **all of you**, I thank you for following our goal to treat patients as family and help them reach a healthier level, live longer and with better quality of life.

To **Elliezer** for creating the magic behind the scenes and doing an amazing job with the cameras, editing and the cover designs of the #AskDrA Books.

To **Lula**, for the distribution of the content through the worldwide web helping more and more people by placing the "Show" before their eyes.

To **Brandi**, for the great spirit and energy transmitted to the team and always being available to my patients online and through social media.

To **Nina**, for the coaching and ideas that we have converted into something amazing that have given us the opportunity to help more and more patients struggling with obesity.

To **Rob**, for the help, support and orientation on the science of social media and for being a partner and co-author.

To **Susan**, my right hand, an angel to many of you that have had the privilege to be coordinated by an amazing good-hearted person and a very knowledgeable nurse that has been part of Endobariatric since day one.

Contents

Contents Continued...

Foreword

By: Rob Anspach

Yes…Vol 2. What an incredible, fun journey learning from not only the best weight loss doctor on the planet, but seeing the thousands of lives transformed as a result of the gastric sleeve procedure. It's just so cool to be part of it all.

The first #AskDrA book was a huge success and gave new "sleevers" answers. And so, to help them on their journey to be happy, healthy and thin…this book continues where the first book left off. Even more answers.

My second visit to Piedras Negras Mexico which occurred as Dr. Alvarez and I were wrapping up this book presented me with the opportunity to meet his family. And when I say family I mean his wife, his children, his parents and the whole Endobariatric team. They just all love and respect him.

I got to tag along on "Meet and Greets" and see first-hand how Dr. A. interacts with patients, sharing stories and telling jokes and making patients feel calm and relaxed prior to surgery.

I got invited into the operating room to watch as Dr. A. and the surgical team changed lives. One of those lives that was changed happened to be a band to sleeve conversion which was interesting to watch up close.

What impressed me the most was that everyone in the OR worked together like clockwork. It was as if they were all linked telepathically, they just knew where to go, what to do and when to do it. It was very impressive to say the least.

Dr. A's commitment to his patient family goes above and beyond and that's why I believe this book series is so important. It continues to help each and every patient discover life as a "sleever" and guides them on their weight loss journey.

So as you read Vol. 2 I hope you gain insight and understanding of how your sleeve works for you, appreciate the dedication that Dr. A. and the Endobariatric team has for all patients (past, present and future) and the impact you can make in other's lives.

When you're done reading this book, hand it to a friend who might be struggling with weight related health issues...and you might be that very person who saves their life.

Thanks for reading.

-Rob Anspach, coauthor

Introduction

By: Dr. Guillermo Alvarez

Welcome to Vol. 2 of the #AskDrA book. It's filled me with overwhelming joy to be able to bring you this great information and useful content that was put together from questions asked by sleeve gastrectomy patients from all over the world. Questions that been submitted from every continent and answered every single week.

To think, it all started the 30th of June of 2015, after finishing that day's surgeries and still wearing my scrubs, I stood in front of the flip camera in my office's waiting room. With no external lighting nor microphone, I decided to take the first few questions and begin answering them talking to a camera with a nonexistent audience.

As the weight loss surgery community started to realize and take notice the show suddenly got shared to external websites, Facebook pages, groups, blogs and even weight loss boards. We started to receive positive feedback from the audience and the weight loss surgery community.

After a year and half of episodes, I'm very pleased to see that the show has continued helping so many. As the show has continued we thought of giving you more ways than just YouTube to be able to have this amazing content available. That's where the idea came about of Volume 2. We started to work on the content of more questions from more episodes for you to have and benefit from.

As with Volume 1 we have added short links at the beginning of each chapter to take you directly to that YouTube episode where we talked about those particular questions. My hope is for you to be filled with this great information, and share your successful weight loss story about the gastric sleeve with your friends.

Let me remind you that you can always be part of the show by submitting questions using the hashtag #AskDrA through Facebook, Twitter, Instagram or YouTube or by connecting directly with me on Snapchat (my username is: gmoalvarez).

I hope you make the most out of this book and most importantly out of your procedure.

Dr. Alvarez

Chapter 27

Harmful Foods, Low Energy Levels, Shrinking Shoe Size

"If you follow the rules you won't do any damage to your sleeve."

To watch the #AskDrA Show episode that this chapter is based on, follow along at:
www.bit.ly/AskDrA27

Are there any foods harmful to eat after sleeve surgery?

Are there any harmful foods after your sleeve? The answer is...and I'll actually answer you with another question. "Are there any harmful foods you can eat before your sleeve?" The answer is, "Yes." You can harm your stomach with or without your sleeve. You can harm the inner layer of your stomach by eating too much spicy food, taking too much of certain medications, consuming too much hot sauce, et cetera.

What you can do to prevent any harm to your sleeve is try to not skip meals. Don't eat too much spicy food. Don't drink too many carbonated beverages. And avoid any medications that pertain to the NSAID family.

Other than that, try to do your normal routine and lifestyle that you used to do before surgery. Try to follow your past regimen of food, food that you're used to. The food that you normally have at dinner with your family. If you follow those general rules you won't do any damage to your sleeve.

Why do my levels of energy go down after each meal?

People who experience some low levels of energy right after your meal may be related to a dumping syndrome. This is a syndrome that we've talked before about. When the food goes into your sleeve and empties right away into the first portion of your small intestine, it may require a lot of blood supply to your gut. It drains your energy right away.

Not everybody experiences this. This is the vast minority of the patients, so don't worry about this. This is temporary in the majority of the cases. It goes away. You don't have to worry about it. Nothing happens. You won't pass out. You just take a nap, wait a while, and as you'll notice, it just passes.

Can feet shrink after losing weight?

Yeah. We see that your feet do shrink. Your feet do shrink along with everything all over. Remember when you have weight-loss surgery, the way you lose the weight is generalized. You lose weight in your fingers, your toes, your arms, legs, belly and everywhere else. Yep, your shoes will become loose. And, it's expected because you're not just going to be losing just 5 or 10 pounds. You're going to be losing 20, 30, 40, 50, 100, 150 pounds.

This weight loss, generalized, affects practically every little corner of your body, and you do lose sizes from your feet. It's expected, and don't worry about it. It's just something normal to deal with in patients that are going to be losing the weight.

Chapter 28

Nausea, Soft Food Phase, Pregnancy

"Follow your doctor's orders. If you do something different, you may end up with a leak, or a complication, it's not worth it."

To watch the #AskDrA Show episode that this chapter is based on, follow along at:
www.bit.ly/AskDrA28

What makes me feel nauseated after eating or drinking? I'm not pregnant, and I'm not a new sleever.

If you didn't experience any nausea the first few weeks or months down the road, and all of a sudden, you get a little bit of nausea, the vast majority of cases is that your sleeve is upset. Your sleeve is swollen or you've got some inflammation in your sleeve, and that is due to something you ate. Maybe you skipped meals, you drank carbonated beverages or alcohol, or ate spicy food... you did something that triggered this inflammation or this swollen tissue. What you need to do, and I said this many times before, is do a round of antacids. Do it for some time, and that should definitely bring that swollen tissue down, and that nausea should disappear.

Can I start soft food phase earlier than supposed to?

No, and this very important for you to understand. You need to follow the guidelines to the T, and you will not have any issues, whatsoever. Follow your doctor's orders. If you do something different, you may end up with a leak, or a complication, it's not worth it. If you've been good for seven, ten days and you want to start your solids but you haven't finished your soft food regimen, it's not worth it, believe me. If you earn yourself a leak, you'll end up back into the hospital, back to the OR, drains all over place, and nothing to eat for weeks. Come on, it's not worth it. Follow the guidelines. You'll be just fine, and after that sleeve heals it's downhill from there. Keep focused. It's the last diet you'll ever do in your life. I promise you.

Can we carry on a pregnancy safely with a sleeve?

Pregnancy after the sleeve is very common. Actually, if you go to YouTube and look for the playlist, "Pregnancy After Sleeve Surgery" you should be able to bring up at least two of my videos. One is a FAQ video and the other one, is Kathryn from Las Vegas, she does a little bit of talking about her pregnancy. Can you get pregnant after your sleeve? Yes. Can you get pregnant right away? Yes, you can. You shouldn't. It's not recommended. I would recommend you wait at least 12 months so that your weight is stabilized. We get a lot of patients from the OBGYNs that are referred to us because of infertility, because of PCOS, or a combination, and they get pregnant right away. "I've never gotten pregnant. Come on, doctor, I've tried for years. It's not going to work," and then they're knocking on my door, three, four months out from surgery. "I'm pregnant. Now what?" Once you start losing weight, fertility in women sky-rises.

Please take care not to get pregnant those first 12 months. Believe me, your body's going to go under a big transformation, getting smaller and smaller, and at the same time, your body's trying to create this new being inside you, so it's not optimal. Once you get pregnant down the road, you'll carry a very good and healthy pregnancy. Last year I had a patient who already stabilized. She got pregnant, she had triplets. The babies are fine, and she was fine, and everything was good. The answer is, you can get pregnant. You'll have to take your maternal vitamins and the vitamins suggested by your OBGYN. Just don't get pregnant right away.

Chapter 29

Protein Intake, Men Vs. Women, Air Travel, Artificial Sweeteners

"Remember that the goal of the pre op diet is to shrink your liver for the surgery."

To watch the #AskDrA Show episode that this chapter is based on, follow along at:
www.bit.ly/AskDrA29

Why is it easier for men to complete the liquid and protein intake than for women?

Men versus women. Normally men have a little bit more capacity. It's easier for them to have a little bit more fluid, protein or shake intake. Right away, after surgery, why? Normally because men have a slightly larger sleeve because it's a little longer. The diameter of the sleeve is exactly the same thing for men and women but they're a little longer with men so that way their capacity is slightly bigger. That's why men struggle less than women right after surgery.

How much time do we have to wait to travel by air?

Travel by plane, you can get on a plane 2 or 3 days after surgery with no problem. Most of our patients travel from coast to coast, around the US, Canada or from other continents. Vast majority of our patients are medical tourism patients, they fly to our center and they get back on a plane 3 days after surgery with no problems. Now, there are a lot of myths out there that if the pressurized cabin of a plane will affect the pressure in your sleeve. Will it blow up in the air? All these just myths. They're all false. Please don't pay any attention to that. You won't have any issues. We've done this for years and we have not had any patient blow up in the air.

Can we have Splenda in our liquid pre and post operation diet?

Using Splenda or artificial sweeteners before surgery, the answer is yes and yes. Using it before surgery reduces the amount of calories you're in-taking per day and that will shrink your liver a lot more. Remember that the goal of the pre op diet is to shrink your liver for the surgery. Using Splenda or artificial sweeteners right after surgery I don't recommend because you actually need regular sugar. You need some carbs to get a good energy level, to feel good. Otherwise you'll feel drained, you'll feel tired, you may feel you may have some headaches. Right after surgery I do want you to use a little bit of sugar. And use juices with regular sugar and fructose. Months after surgery you may switch back to the artificial sweeteners because that lowers your carb intake and it helps you lose weight faster and at a steady pace. The answer is yes, it's just a matter of time when to use it.

Chapter 30

Drinking Too Fast or Slow, Feeling Hungry, Losing Weight Pace

"As the day's go by, the swollen tissue goes away and the fluids will go down nicely."

To watch the #AskDrA Show episode that this chapter is based on, follow along at: www.bit.ly/AskDrA30

I'm eight-days post operation and when I drink four ounces of liquid I don't feel restriction, why?

Right after surgery, you may feel some restriction to liquids which is normal because the sleeve is so swollen. After day two, day three, day four you may notice that this restriction may be less and it may be gone even after day five, day six or even day seven. This is totally normal. This may be even sooner, day two, day three, you're drinking fluids nicely. Don't focus on this as a restriction. Fluids need to go down. They need to go through the sleeve. Look at it as a pipe, as a drain. Fluids will go down through that drain, through that pipe, nicely without restriction.

The reason you have restriction right after surgery is because the sleeve is so swollen you'll get restriction to even fluids at that point. As the day's go by, the swollen tissue goes away and the fluids will go down nicely. That is why we progress with clear liquids, then we jump to thicker stuff which is full liquids and then soft foods and so on. This is totally normal and expected. Restriction right away, even to fluids, then it goes away after day three, day four. Then, we'll jump to full liquids after day seven, so on and so forth but that's totally normal.

I'm eight weeks post operation and today I feel hungry. Is it normal?

Feeling hungry after surgery? Some people, right after surgery may notice it. Talking about the swollen tissue right after the sleeve. The swollen tissue of the sleeve, your brain will detect it as hunger. You'll say, wait a minute, I thought the surgery was to put that hunger away, now I'm hungry right after surgery. What's going on? Or at week eight or at week three, etc. The swollen tissue of the sleeve may produce this hunger sensation. Be sure you're taking your antacid right after surgery. Follow your doctor's guidelines as the swollen tissue will go away with this acid blocker and the sensation will go away. These patients, we give them a round of anti-acids. It could be Prilosec, Omeprazole, some other acid blocker. We do it for quite a few weeks, maybe four weeks and the acid goes away and guess what? That hunger sensation goes away too. What you're really experiencing as hunger is actually just the swollen tissues, the acid production right after surgery.

What is a good average weight loss for a newly sleeved patient?

What is a good losing pace? Answer, it varies. It varies from patient to patient because everybody is different. If you sleeve a 400-pound patient versus a 300-pound patient verses a 200-pound, it's very different. The 400-pound patient will lose more because he or she needs to lose more. It will come off faster. Also another tendency is exercise activity or activity level. This will speed up your metabolism, will speed up the losing pace of your body. To give you more or less of an idea, right after surgery, the average good losing pace is a half a pound to a pound and a half or even two pounds per week. That will vary from half a pound to two pounds per week. That's a good pace. Remember that I'm not talking about stalls. We've talked about stalls before. Stalls are normal. Stalls are needed. They don't come into this average weekly losing pace, all right.

Number one, focus. Number two, stay on the guidelines. Number three, don't focus on the numbers because the weight will come off sooner or later. Keep doing what you need to do. Lower your carb intake, increase exercise activity and you'll be just fine.

Chapter 31

Snacking, Protein Consumption, Tenderness At The Incision Site

"The body can only process so much protein at a time. So, it's better to spread it out throughout the day."

To watch the #AskDrA Show episode that this chapter is based on, follow along at: www.bit.ly/AskDrA31

What do you recommend as an in between meal snack?

Snacking with your sleeve. As you know people with a sleeve normally tend to eat a mid-morning or mid afternoon snack, so it depends on what your goal is and what you're working on. If you're working with a low calorie or a low carb option, my "go to" choice is celery sticks. Celery sticks contain good fiber, they are low carb and have a really good amount of a fluid. Oh and you can always change the dipping dressing you want to accompany your celery.

As to fruit...my choice is apples and peaches. If you're looking for more choices, you can search online for "healthy snacking to work with your sleeve".

Can I consume all my proteins in the morning or is it better to stretch the consumption throughout the day?

Like you, I've heard it several ways. But here's the thing...the body can only process so much protein at a time. So, it's better to spread it out throughout the day, specifically when you are doing some type of workout. Remember that the base of maintaining muscle is to avoid losing muscle while only losing the fat. You need good protein and exercise. When people exercise what they do is they take a portion of protein before their workout, and then a portion of protein after the workout.

Splitting your protein will give you the best muscle development. It'll take care of that muscle. It won't burn muscle. Then let's say you don't want to worry about the protein. You just want to get it over with. You take a big muscle milk protein shake which is sixty grams in the morning. You're done. You think you don't have to worry about it throughout the day. Now you won't starve. But by the end of the day you may feel deprived and hungry. So the ideal course of action is just spread it out throughout the day. It'll be much better.

Your body will assimilate it much better, and it'll also help you with protecting your muscles. If you're working out please, please spread it out throughout the day and get that protein in close to your workout. It'll be much better.

My scars always hurt. Is this normal?

We call this incision pain. You may experience it, some do and some don't. In our practice if you do experience incision pain it'll come from the largest left incision. The days following a surgery you will notice patients, or even yourself if you just underwent the procedure, holding their hand just a bit left of their belly button area. Why is that? Because there's tenderness on that side. It's where we pulled that big chunk of stomach out.

It may vary from practice to practice because some surgeons may take that piece of stomach out through the center incision, but the vast majority of practices will go out through the left side. That pain is completely normal unless of course you are months or years down the road. Just make sure you don't have a hernia or something developed there. In our practice we use a big stitch that runs right through the abdominal wall and comes right out we do this to prevent hernias down the road. That means that our percentage of hernias developing after surgery is dropped down to the minimum.

Like I stated, it depends on every practice. I tell my

patients I prefer you're a little sore on that left side so no hernias developed down the road.

Chapter 32

Weight Stalls, Eating and Drinking, Counting Carbs

"Make it a process. Don't jump from not counting carbs to under 30 right away because you'll go crazy."

To watch the #AskDrA Show episode that this chapter is based on, follow along at:
www.bit.ly/AskDrA32

I have lost only 2 pounds in 4 weeks. Is that normal?

It varies from patient to patient. Put your mind at ease. You're doing good. The average losing pace, and we talked about this in Chapter 30, the amount of...the losing pace varies from patient to patient. The more you have to lose the more you'll lose right away and then it will stall and then you'll lose again and then it will stall and then you'll lose again. That is normal. If you hit a stall and you've only lost 2 pounds in 4 weeks. It's normal. Don't freak out. These stalls are normal. Remember I've got some videos out there on my YouTube channel just type in "weight stalls" or "weight stalls Dr. Alvarez" and YouTube will show you that video.

These stalls are normal. They're needed. Your body needs to adapt and get used to this new weight then it will restart the weight loss again.

Number 1- the pace is different on every patient.
Number 2- weight stalls or plateaus are normal.
Number 3- patience, exercise, and keep focused.

Those are the keys right there.

Does drinking and eating stretch out your sleeve?

The answer is no, but eating and drinking at the same time may give you a kind of weird or uncomfortable sensation. It won't burst your sleeve. It doesn't expand your sleeve. It just feels weird. The fluid is competing for space with that food in your newly crafted sleeve and it feels kind of uncomfortable.

To avoid that sensation, don't drink anything 30 minutes before eating. Then you may start drinking 30-45 minutes after you finished eating. Follow this tip you'll avoid this uncomfortable sensation.

Now, not everybody gets that sensation. Again it varies from patient to patient.

How many grams a day of carbs should we be taking? 30, 40, I've even heard people say up to 50.

So if you're counting carbs what amount of intake should you be under to be losing weight? Well, a vast majority of my patients are under 30 grams.

But it takes time. If you start off and can keep it under 30, great…but it's kind of difficult, I've done it. I know.

Start off at a level that you can manage. If you start at 100 work your way down. Then you can do the next step and be under 50. Then the ultimate, you want to keep it under 30. Make it a process. Don't jump from not counting carbs to under 30 right away because you'll go crazy and want to go kill Dr. Alvarez. Don't do that.

Take it easy. Take it slow. Try to keep it under 30. If you're doing under 30 just keep it at that pace and your fat is just going to be melting off. You'll like it.

Chapter 33

Spinning Classes, Tea & Coffee, Blood Loss

"Everything that's fluid counts as part of your daily goal or fluid intake."

To watch the #AskDrA Show episode that this chapter is based on, follow along at:
www.bit.ly/AskDrA33

How often should a four weeks out sleever go to spinning class per week?

Let's talk about exercise in general. Remember that if everything was a success with your sleeve 15 days out from surgery you can start doing some walking, get on an elliptical machine, get on a treadmill and walk for 15-20 minutes but don't do more than that. There's more than enough time for the rest of your life to exercise. Don't try to kill yourself doing exercise right away.

I've told patients, and you've probably seen this before on my previous videos...that exercise is like brushing your teeth. You don't brush your teeth for two hours straight. You brush your teeth several times a day, a low amount of time. This is the same thing with exercise. It's more the frequency and making it a habit than trying to kill yourself doing an hour and half, two hours, three hours of exercise just because you're eager to lose weight. No, no, no. Patience! Time is the key here. All right? So make sure you are taking it easy, 10 to 15 minutes. And you're all set.

After four weeks you can increase your intensity. You can start doing spinning classes easily. You can pretty much do anything at this point. Go easy with the weight lifting though.

Does decaf coffee or tea count as water intake?

The answer is yes.

All of that counts as fluid intake. I'm going to throw in this tip right here, this is key...remember to keep a diary, a log on what you are in-taking and how often. I have this cool water bottle. It's clear and flat and I can take it anywhere, I fill up it twice a day. That water is what I need to intake per day. I want you to do the same thing. I want you to keep a log of what you're in-taking. It's very important because otherwise you don't know. You don't know how much you're in-taking. Back to the question, back to the answer, the answer is yes. Everything that's fluid counts as part of your daily goal or fluid intake.

What is the average of blood loss during a surgery?

It's not that frequent of a question, but it's a good question. I sometimes hear that question here in my office when my patient is right in front of me and asking me how much blood loss should I expect? With our technique, I tell patients that you'll probably bleed more from the blood work that's going to be drawn out of you for the testing than the surgery itself. I'm not kidding. At least with us, that's our average. Our average is not even a gauze of soaked blood. That's less than five millimeters per surgery. Of course there can be, talking in general, circumstances, that we've encountered like a big hiatal hernia and one of the vessels starts to bleed then you stop it and then there's a little bit more blood, but on average, a normal situation is you'll bleed more from the blood work than the surgery itself. Pretty cool, huh?

Chapter 34

Changing Taste Buds, How To Gain Weight, Low Carb Diet

"If you wish to gain a little weight simply increase your carb intake."

To watch the #AskDrA Show episode that this chapter is based on, follow along at:
www.bit.ly/AskDrA34

So many foods taste different after surgery. I wonder if this is permanent?

The taste buds are known to change. This is not common on everybody. This happens to a very low percentage of patients, but it is common. This is just temporary, everything returns to normal. Remember that with the sleeve that portion of your stomach that produces some hormones inside your gut is also adjusting. Don't freak out. This is totally normal. It is not permanent, nor does this happen to everybody.

What do you suggest I should do if I want to gain a little weight?

That is not a common question, right? But if you want to gain more weight all you have to do is increase your carb intake. It's quite simple. Increasing your carb intake will make you stall at a certain weight, or if you increase it more, your daily intake of carbs, it will make you gain weight. Plus, carbs are the easiest thing that go down the Sleeve, and it will make you gain weight. No other thing, neither protein nor fat. Your sleeve gets full much quicker with carbs. So if you wish to gain a little weight simply increase your carb intake. That's the best advice.

Can you explain to everybody why it's so important to follow a low-carb, low-sugar, and high-protein meals after surgery?

It's a really good question, so let me tell you why. Carbs have everything to do related to weight loss, and the Gastric Sleeve patient, so I always push low-carb, low-carb, low-carb. Except initially right after the Sleeve, where I push high-carb. Look for the sugar you need it, because it'll give you energy and make you feel good. You need the energy, because your brain, your heart, your kidneys work, or function with sugar or carbs. Instead of feeling weak, or light headed, or with a headache right after surgery I tell you to consume some carbs, because you're still going to be doing a low amount of calories per day, you're still going to be losing weight, and that's fine.

Once you start eating, and you're a few months out, I always push patients to go low-carb. Why? Because going low-carb will kick in a metabolic process, a chemical process in your body, because your brain, your heart, your kidneys need to function with carbs. Your body will look for these carbs, and since you're not putting carbs in, your body will actually make these carbs for you. Where? It grabs it from your stored fat. Your body grabs it from there, takes it to the liver, converts it to carbs, and you can use it, so your body functions perfectly fine. Bring it to low-carb it'll give you the best weight loss down the road.

Why the high protein? Because protein maintains muscle, so it's important to maintain a good muscle mass. That way you're losing fat, and not the muscle. We want you to lose weight from your stored fat, and not that much from the muscle. To protect the muscle two things: protein intake, exercise.

Chapter 35

Myth, Smells, Energy Drinks, Weight Lifting

"Please, don't start trying to lift heavy weights. You need to go slow and build it up, as with all exercise."

To watch the #AskDrA Show episode that this chapter is based on, follow along at:
www.bit.ly/AskDrA35

My Aunt had 50% of her stomach removed 40 years ago and every time she eats she has to run to the bathroom to poop. Is that a risk of the gastric sleeve?

Let's bring in a little bit of history here. The gastric sleeve is a relatively new procedure. It was performed by Dr. Gagner in 1999. By the year 2001 it was being done laparoscopically, and it's been done that way ever since. Forty years ago it wasn't a gastric sleeve. This is a relatively new procedure, but there is this myth that if you eat after a gastric sleeve surgery, you will go poop right away, and that's totally not true. That does not happen. That's a myth. Remember, this is totally different. Gastric sleeve surgery versus a gastric bypass or a duodenal switch where rapid gastric emptying may occur, commonly referred as "dumping syndrome" may occur.

The issues related to the Aunt's procedure are related more to mal-absorption procedures like a gastric bypass, duodenal switch, but not as much or not at all regarding the gastric sleeve surgery.

Is it normal that the smell of certain items provoke nausea?

Put your mind at ease. It's uncommon for people to experience nausea caused by certain smells. Yes, certain tastes may change, and we talked about that in a previous chapter, but smells, nope not that common. Remember that these symptoms are usually just temporary. They'll go away. It's probably just a day or two and then they'll probably go away, so don't worry about that.

Are energy drinks okay to have during pre-operation diet?

Okay, bottom line here's 4 reasons why I have to say NO! Number one, I don't like them. Number two, I don't recommend them. Number three, they're not good for you. Number four, just don't use them. Let me tell you why. Energy drinks have a whole bunch of "stuff" in there (It's easier to say "stuff" then chemicals, preservatives, artificial flavorings, sugars, etc.). Why not just switch it to something like water or tea or unsweetened tea, or something like that? Energy drinks will give you energy. Yeah, that's true. It's got a whole bunch of that "stuff" that will make your energy level rise, but the downside, the crash won't make you feel good. I would stay away from them.

How long does it take to start lifting heavy weights after weight loss surgery?

Heavy weights, 30 days is practically the amount of time you need to wait after surgery so you can start lifting some weights. Please, don't start trying to lift 150, 200, 250, 300 pounds. You need to go slow and build it up as with all exercise. Get yourself a trainer. Tell them you've had the gastric sleeve surgery. Tell them you've had weight loss surgery. Most of them know about the procedure, and they'll know how to train you accordingly. They'll take you slow with many reps and then start adding up some weights.

Chapter 36

Converting The Sleeve, Hours of Sleep, Have I Had Surgery

"Keep track of how many hours of sleep you're getting, because it's important for your body to recover."

To watch the #AskDrA Show episode that this chapter is based on, follow along at:
www.bit.ly/AskDrA36

It is possible to turn the sleeve into gastric bypass?

Can you switch from a gastric sleeve to a gastric bypass? The answer is yes. It's quite simple to do so, and it is reserved normally for high BMI patients, higher BMIs than 52. You can convert your sleeve into bypass or you can convert your sleeve into a duodenal switch. Both options are available. We are doing some other analysis with other procedures called single anastomosis.

If you're thinking of converting a sleeve to gastric bypass or duodenal switch, please make sure that you analyze what is going on and why you're not losing weight. Normally, the vast majority of our patients, it's because there's something that you're not doing, or you're not following certain guidelines. Do a diary of what you're eating, if you want to use an application on your phone you can always use My Fitness Pal. It helps you track, log and analyze what's going on. Maybe it's just your bad eating habits and that's not helping you. If you wish to convert your sleeve into a bypass or duodenal switch you can, that's your decision but don't do it just because you've got 20, 30 pounds to go. No.

Those 20, 30 pounds is because you're doing something wrong and you can actually get back on track quite simple. Watch my videos! We talk about that a lot, okay?

How many hours of sleep at night is healthy for a sleeve patient?

It's very important, because a gastric sleeve patient goes under quite a bit of transformation, your body needs some sleep. I would recommend at least seven hours of sleep. Keep track of how many hours of sleep you're getting, because it's important for your body to recover. Getting at least seven hours is good. Eight is fantastic! Less than six, beware because you will develop a chronic fatigue because your body's going through a lot of changes. You need to sleep. Keep track.

Have I (Dr. Alvarez) had the sleeve surgery?

No, I really wish I did. I did lose about 40 pounds though. I lost it by doing a low-carb diet. If you want that diet, I have it. I actually wrote it down myself.

My patients who belong to our private Facebook group have access to that diet, but I can always send it out to anybody. I lost the weight and pretty much kept it off. Of course, I'm a big cyclist. Whenever I can I get back on my bike I go for the distance. You can also do it. Of course patients who have the sleeve get the most out of it doing a low-carb diet down the road. The results are just phenomenal.

Chapter 37

Fat and Protein, Bruising, Numbness

"Count your carbs then bring them down under 50 and then ultimately under 30 and you will be a burning fat machine."

To watch the #AskDrA Show episode that this chapter is based on, follow along at:
www.bit.ly/AskDrA37

How many fats and proteins should we be aiming for?

I really don't want you to worry about how much fat to consume after surgery. What I want you to focus on how much protein to consume after surgery which is at least 1 gram per every 2.2 pounds of ideal body weight you should have. If you use the metric system, it's 1 gram per every kilogram of ideal weight you should be weighing. Ideally, between 70 to 80 to 90 grams of protein per day is really good. More than enough to preserve your muscle, that way you don't burn that muscle while you're losing the weight.

We didn't mention carbs in that question but I want to throw it in. Lower your carb intake once you've crossed the diet phases (phase 1, phase 2, phase 3) and once you start eating solid foods 2 or 3 months down the road. You can start cutting down your carbs slowly, slowly bringing them down to 100 grams per day. Count your carbs then bring them down under 50 and then ultimately under 30 and you will be a burning fat machine. You'll be doing amazing because you're going to be having the restriction of your gastric sleeve and you're going to be having your metabolic process burning fat. You'll love the process.

Is it normal to have bruises around my belly button after surgery?

Bruising after surgery? Yes! Around the belly button may be related directly to the surgery. Let me tell you why, because we normally enter through a tiny incision above the belly button. Unfortunately, we don't see the tiny vessels underneath throughout the fat tissue and that may have bruised a bit and that bruising, with gravity, may come down toward your belly button. When the bruising happens right after surgery it's nothing to be worried about. Now bruising months after surgery I would recommend you get checked. Make sure your blood levels are good. And your CBC, platelet level and iron level are all good too.

Is it normal to have numbness with the sleeve?

This is kind of frequent. There is a small, very small percentage of patients that may experience some numbness in a certain area in their body. Sometimes legs, sometimes thighs. This is not that frequent but we do see it. Don't freak out. I would suggest you check your vitamin levels. Taking vitamin B complex will help recover the sensation. Don't get concerned. Everything will reverse 100% once you start taking the B complex as the weeks go by.

Chapter 38

Tanning, Switching Band To Sleeve, Mood Swings

"Some people just don't understand the psychological aspect of doing a pre-op diet. But it helps you stay mentally focused on losing weight."

To watch the #AskDrA Show episode that this chapter is based on, follow along at:
www.bit.ly/AskDrA38

Can I tan in a tanning bed if I am two weeks post operation?

Yes, you can, but I would recommend you wait. I tell my patients, "You want a tan, go ahead and do so, just maybe cover your incisions up with the Band-Aid or a surgical tape, something to cover them up." Why? Because if you tan without covering the incisions, the pigmentation around those incisions will get darker and down the road will look different. Unless you cover them up, don't tan. If you're covering them up, that's fine. After 6 months, you can tan all together. You won't have any issues down the road.

Can I have my band removal surgery and the gastric sleeve surgery in the same day?

Switching from a band to a sleeve, can it be done in one step? Yes, but and there's a big but here...you can get it done in one step if it's safe. Safety is number one priority. Switching from a band to a sleeve can be done if we go in, we see the band is lying nicely, minimum scar tissue, minimal adhesions, and we can break this down, take the band system off and we can convert that into a sleeve in one step. Perfect. Sometimes we go in there and either because the band's been in there too long or the original surgeon was messy and created chaos or there's lots of scar tissue. There's a lot of factors that go in, even the type of band you received.

There are some bands that cause less scar tissue than others. All these factors come into play and give us an end result of scar tissue and adhesions. Now, sometimes we go in and it's just like the band was installed yesterday. We can take the band system out and we convert that into a sleeve in one step, no problem. Sometimes we go in there, it looks like a bomb exploded. It's chaos and we need to go get that band system out, and we need to wait. We need to wait because we need to let the stomach settle down, let the scar tissue calm down, no band there provoking more inflammation and swollen tissue. After a few months, we come back without that band being there and the stomach is all set and prepared. We go in and we convert that into sleeve.

How often is the switch? It's about 70/30. Seventy percent get that band to sleeve in one step; the other thirty percent have to wait. But I do tell patients, remember, this is something that you can't control, I don't control it, or your previous surgeon can't control it. That's how the band is...and how your body reacts to a foreign substance inside you. Everybody reacts to a foreign body differently. Sometimes it's bad; sometimes it's slight and we can convert that in one step, all right?

Is it common to have problems with my emotions after the surgery?

Not common, but if present, it may be related to several factors. One is lack of carbs and lack of energy. Maybe you had a quite a bit of rough recovery, it happens, and a minority of our patients experience it too. This can be easily addressed or can be easily avoided. One major thing: doing that pre-op diet well gets your body adjusted before surgery. Some people just don't understand the psychological aspect of doing a pre-op diet. They think it's just because I want to give them a hard time or their surgeon wants to give them a hard time. It's not like that.

It's because it creates a body of physical adaptation to a lower amount of calories per day, but also the mindset is very important and it helps you down the road after surgery. If you don't do this correctly, you may have these mood swings because you're lacking calories, because you're lacking some carbs, or sugar, or something. If you do the pre-op diet before, then it's a piece of cake. You'll be adapted psychologically and physically. Keep focused and be aware of what's going on if you're having these mood swings so you can address it.

Chapter 39

Muscle Cramps, Solid Foods, High Impact Sports

"Focus on hydration as your number one thing."

To watch the #AskDrA Show episode that this chapter is based on, follow along at: www.bit.ly/AskDrA39

What can I do if I'm experiencing cramps in my legs and hands?

Muscle cramps or muscle spasms are not normal so you need to figure out what is causing the muscle spasms. There are two causes of muscle spasms. The first one is dehydration. That's the number one cause in gastric sleeve patients that are struggling to get hydrated the first few days or weeks after surgery. Now as the swollen tissue from surgery comes down, you'll be able to intake more water at a time. Staying hydrated will make those muscle spasms or cramps go away.

The other thing is a lack of potassium. This you'll have to check with your doctor, get some blood drawn to make sure your potassium is at a good level.

Most of our patients have high blood pressure and diabetes, especially high blood pressure and some medications will effect potassium levels. There are also some medications that may cause you to go to pee more frequently and may lose a little bit of potassium at that time. Those patients may have some muscle cramps more commonly than other patients. Take home message is to focus on hydration as the number one thing. If you're taking some other medication especially or specifically for high blood pressure, check with your doctor.

Can I eat solid food the night before a surgery?

This answer may vary from patient to patient or surgical practice to surgical practice. In our practice, you may not take any solid food the day before surgery. A vast majority of the patients depending on the BMI will be required to do a pre-op diet. This helps at the time of surgery to, number one, shrink the liver. Number two to have enough space to perform your surgery. And number three, it gets your mind set for the psychological aspect of losing weight and that you're prepared mentally, that after surgery you're going to be doing a post-op diet. You're going to be just fine.

This is our practice. Check with your doctor. In our practice, 99.9% of our patients don't eat any solid food the day before surgery or days before surgery because they're doing a pre-op diet based on liquids.

If I did my surgery this summer, can I play football in August?

Let's talk about high impact sports and their recovery time. In this case, the patient is asking that if they get surgery done in June or July will he be able or be ready for football season in August. High impact sports like football, boxing, karate, martial arts, etcetera, may take up to a month to recover completely. I tell patients yes you may do that, but after thirty days. Start slowly after fifteen days. Start walking, exercising and build up your cadence from there up until your thirty days is out. You're able to pretty much do any type of exercise, even high impact sports.

Chapter 40

Sensations, Low Carb Diet, Creatine & Sleeve Pillows

"I tell patients that every single symptom they feel right after sleeve surgery is totally normal and just temporary. Those sensations will go away."

To watch the #AskDrA Show episode that this chapter is based on, follow along at:
www.bit.ly/AskDrA40

How long will the feeling of everything traveling down your sleeve last?

That sensation or feeling of the food going down through your sleeve is only temporary. I tell patients that every single symptom they feel right after sleeve surgery is totally normal and just temporary. Those sensations will go away. Again, totally normal. But, not everybody feels those sensations. Number one, its normal. Number two, its temporary. Normally lasts two or three days after the procedure and then it goes away.

Now, if this is a sensation that comes after a few weeks out or after a few months out, that's totally different. Maybe your sleeve is swollen. Be sure to look at my video, "The Swollen Sleeve".

Type in "Swollen Sleeve Dr. Alvarez" on YouTube and be sure to watch that video.

It's probably just swollen and it's simple to take care of it.

My husband follows a high protein and low carb diet, but immediately after eating he gets tired. What can he do?

So whenever you do a low carb diet or high protein low carb diet, the first few days, there is an adaptation period that people may feel some symptoms like being weak, fatigued, maybe a headache, maybe some dizziness. All these new sensations is actually your body adapting to your new diet program. Your body kicks in with the process which forces your liver to release stored glycogen which creates the added carbs in your body needs. Once it kicks in, those sensations of weakness and fatigue go away.

The best advice is to start counting carbs by lowering them over time. Start at under one hundred first and then under fifty and then ultimately under thirty per day. It's not that drastic and you won't have these symptoms long. Once your body adapts those symptoms go away.

Is it okay to take creatine after the surgery?

Yes, you can take some supplements including creatine and whey protein for building muscle. But I would wait at least 30 days after surgery before taking them. These products are designed to help with muscle building and I tell all my patients to limit the heavy lifting after surgery. Thirty days out...you're good. The supplements won't affect your sleeve so there is no worries there, but wait to take them until you're healed from surgery.

Chapter 41

Iron, Essential Oils, Sauna and Stretched Sleeve

"Please do not compare the amount of food you intake months or years down the road to the first few weeks to months after surgery."

To watch the #AskDrA Show episode that this chapter is based on, follow along at:
www.bit.ly/AskDrA41

Do you need to wait to take your iron pill when drinking milk or eating yogurt?

Iron as a supplement is good. Normally taken by women, that have a tendency to have anemia because they've got some bleeding or other issue. If you're told by a physician to take iron, the best way and ideal way to take iron is with an empty stomach.

But keep in mind…iron is aggressive and rough on an empty stomach specifically on the gastric sleeve. Some people would say, "Well, how about if I take it with a glass of milk?" The thing is, anything that contains calcium like milk or a drinkable yogurt or anything like that may alter the absorption of iron.

My suggestion is take your antacid in the morning possibly at noon then in the evening and if you take your iron on an empty stomach you're covered. So yes, if you take iron with anything that is dairy that has some calcium which they do, your iron supplement will not be absorbed the way it should.

Is it okay to use essential oils in your water?

We have this new tendency of essential oils now that can be added in and on food, in water, to other liquids and used for rubbing. The answer is...yes, you can use essential oils. It won't interfere at all with the healing process or phase 1 clear liquids or phase 2 or from thereon. All safe.

How soon after being sleeved can I get back to enjoying sauna time?

Okay so here's the deal...I'm not worried at all about your incisions after seven or ten days going into a sauna for enjoying the heat and the relaxing effects, I'm worried about you getting dehydrated. Number one thing here is avoiding dehydration. Do NOT enjoy a sauna the first few weeks after your surgery, you'll get dehydrated. You can only intake so much water fluids at a time with the sleeve the first few weeks and I would at least wait at least a month when you're able to intake more fluids at a time. Your urine is clear, not concentrated and after those 30 days, your incisions are all nicely healed and you're clear there, so wait at least 30 days. Before that, you're risking it, risking dehydration because let's face it gets kind of hot in a sauna.

If you get off track and your sleeve stretches, will it retract and go back to its original restriction?

Can you get back on track if you fell off the wagon because you think your sleeve is stretched out. Well, there's no way to know that your sleeve is stretched out if you haven't had an upper endoscopy or barium swallow to see the anatomy of your stomach or your current sleeve. If you think that the sleeve stretches out because you're eating a little bit more or you're eating more compared to the first few weeks or months after surgery...the answer is No. Because the first few weeks after surgery or even after a couple of months, you're at the maximum restriction of the gastric sleeve and from there on, as the swollen tissue starts to come down, you're going to be noticing that you're able to intake more at a time.

Please do not compare the amount of food you

intake months or years down the road to the first few weeks to months after surgery. You'll notice that you're able to intake much less amount of food than before surgery. But remember that the first few weeks to months after your surgery, that's the maximum point of restriction, it's not fair to compare that to years down the road with your sleeve and saying your sleeve has stretched because you got more capacity.

To say, it's stretched, you need to have some studies done to see actually if it is stretched, how was your technique performed, what type of bougie did they use to create or perform your surgery? There's all these factors, all right? Don't just say, "Well, my sleeve is stretched out and I fell off the wagon." You can always get back on track.

If you feel you've fallen off wagon, then you need to lower your carb intake. That's the easiest way for weight loss surgery patients to get back on track. Number one, lower the carb intake and number two, physical activity. Please do not leave everything to your sleeve. Remember your sleeve is a tool. You need to work with it so please do not let your sleeve do all the work. You need to put some effort there.

Chapter 42

Staples, Cutting Hair & Coming Alone For Your Weight Loss Surgery

"The staples we use are made out of titanium, they are 100% biocompatible and will not produce an allergic reaction."

To watch the #AskDrA Show episode that this chapter is based on, follow along at:
www.bit.ly/AskDrA42

What metal are the staples made of and what companies manufactures the staples?

A very common question that I get sometimes is, "Doctor what type of material are the staples made of because I'm kind of concerned. I'm allergic to nickel." Or maybe they get a rash. Remember that the staples used for surgery are made out of titanium. It's the same material used for knee replacement, hip replacement, etc. Why titanium? Because titanium is the only material known to mankind that is 100% biocompatible. What this means is it will not produce an allergic reaction. Put your mind at ease. It won't cause any issues at all.

Now there are two major manufacturers of staples. One is Covidien, which is now owned by Medtronic. The other brand is Ethicon Endo-surgery, which is Johnson & Johnson. Those are the two major brands used world-wide. There are some other brands out there. We don't even bother to mention nor even use. Other manufacturers do not have the safety requirements that need to be implemented for our patients, so we don't mess around with those companies. I don't even recommend them. I won't even bother mentioning them. Two companies with top quality materials, Johnson & Johnson, which is Ethicon Endo-surgery and Covidien, which is now Medtronic. Those two are top notch and safety centered and great material for your sleeves.

Should I cut my hair before surgery so the hair loss is not too noticeable?

Well, I wouldn't worry about the hair loss. You may have some hair thinning. We've talked about this before. There is a lot of factors that go into play; nutrition, supplements and body transformation. The vast majority of patients don't experience hair loss. If you like your hair long, keep it that way. If it thins out, if you want to cut it down the road, well, it's a personal preference. There's no medical reason to actually cut it before surgery.

Will I be okay with no one with me when I go for the surgery?

Well, having surgery or coming to Mexico for surgery by yourself is very common in our practice.

We get a lot of patients who come from the U.S., from coast to coast, Canada and even other continents in the world, that come to our center by themselves. I always ask them before surgery. We talk. I interview them. We go over the health history together and everything. I always ask the patient, would you like me to call somebody back home once we're done or you're in recovery? Some say yes. Some say no. The option is always there. Yeah. It's a common practice. People come down for their surgeries by themselves.

Remember it's a 25, 35-minute surgery, really quick. We're always available to call family members back home. This is not just only for my practice. You'll see this in other practices around the country, it's fairly common.

Chapter 43

Upper Endoscopy, Time Needed Off Work, Cramping Pain After Surgery

"Recovery after sleeve surgery is very quick. And most patients return to their normal routine after just a few days."

To watch the #AskDrA Show episode that this chapter is based on, follow along at:
www.bit.ly/AskDrA43

What is the recommended time frame for an EGD after the surgery?

So let's talk about upper endoscopies and when is it safe to have a study like this done after your sleeve. Don't get me wrong I believe this is a valid procedure. And it can help detect strictures, complications and leaks. The endoscopy can be done immediately right after surgery, although it's not recommended on a normal recovery of a gastric sleeve patient.

Let's say you have a normal sleeve, normal recovery. I wouldn't recommend having an upper endoscopy within the first 6 weeks after surgery. Well, 6 weeks is good but if you can wait at least 6 months, that would be even better. Unless there is a complication or certain indication, your surgeon wants to get it done, otherwise wait 6 weeks, better so 6 months.

How long is it okay to take off of work after the surgery?

How much time do you need off work? If you have a

desk job, 3 to 5 days normally and patients are back to work. Let's say that's the average. Some people need a little bit more. 7 days would be awesome. 10 days is, believe me, more than enough time. Remember, this procedure is done laparoscopically. Tiny, tiny incisions and recovery is fairly quickly. Patients are getting up to go to the restroom 2 to 3 hours after surgery. That same evening, patients are walking up and down the hall. Recovery is very, very quick. It would require a little more extra time if your job requires heavy lifting, otherwise if it's just a desk job, 3 to 5 days.

Every time I eat, I get an almost cramping pain on my left side. What could be that?

So a cramping pain after 10 months is not normal. First of all, check with your doctor and then make sure, that it's your gallbladder. If you don't have your gallbladder, if it's previously taken out, make sure your sleeve is good. Maybe at this point it's a good time to get an upper endoscopy and check your sleeve out, but it's not a common situation to have pain this far out. Normally patients may have this cramping sensation, this pain, the first few days after surgery, which not everybody gets. The first few days, a cramping sensation, once you start doing the ice, once you start doing clear liquids, 2 or 3 days out, and then it disappears. Ten months out, I would check with your surgeon or your doctor just to make sure everything's good. Get an ultrasound of your gallbladder, make sure it's not another issue other than your sleeve.

Chapter 44

Gummies, Mexico, Requirements, Protocols & Converting To A Sleeve

"Your stomach will never ever be the size it was before surgery so keep that in mind. You will never ever have that stomach again."

To watch the #AskDrA Show episode that this chapter is based on, follow along at: www.bit.ly/AskDrA44

Do the gummy vitamins have carbs?

It's a multi-vitamin in gummy form and yes they do have carbs. The amount of carbs they have is minimum. If you're focused on a low carb diet, try to look for an alternative. If your diet is plant based and you're looking for supplementation you can take the gummies because they have a little bit of carbs and that's fine. The most important thing is to take something. If you can take a multi-vitamin, or B12, some calcium and some iron, you're covered, but if you have problems shallowing those supplements, then take the gummies.

What is the difference in cost in Mexico and the States?

The reason is cost. I try to help out as many patients I can and the way I can do that is by practicing in Mexico. Same standards as any U.S. hospital, but cost is less. How much less? In some cases, half the price in the U.S. With some procedures, I heard some hospitals in the States charge from 25 to a crazy $40,000 for a sleeve...and ours is $8900. That includes absolutely everything, all you have to do is put yourself in San Antonio, Texas and we'll pick you up. We have a whole logistic system set up. Hotels are paid, transportation is paid, door to door service. And we make you feel secure and comfortable.

The health system requires a lot in the U.S.A. What are your requirements?

Interesting fact. The healthcare system and the insurance companies in the US have made things so complicated. What they want is not to have to pay for anything. They'll make you jump through hoops, go see a psychologist, go see a nutritionist, make sure you're not crazy, make sure you know what you're getting into. I mean you're an adult, you know that you're obese, you know you want a solution. You're tired, you've done dieting, and yo-yo'ing, you want to take this step.

There are really good clinical trials, studies out there, that compare the U.S. system versus the European system or the Australian system where they don't have to go through all the jumping hoops, cardiologist, internal doctor, internal medicine, nutritionist, psychologist and everything else. They've determined that that is just a waste of time. We'll do a complete blood work panel, we'll do an EKG, chest x-ray, we evaluate you and make sure you're healthy to go into an OR. Then if you're good to go, we perform the surgery, we make sure you're feeling okay and and then we have a special online system that will follow up with you afterwards for a complete year.

I have a lap-band, can it be converted to a sleeve?

Did you know I did a band on my mom? Yep, I placed a band in my mom back in 2006. Back then the band was hot. Everybody wanted one. The marketing of the band was very attractive. The manufacturers gave claims that the band surgery was removable, reversible, adjustable and minimally evasive. They sold people on the idea that surgeons don't cut into your stomach, they don't staple your stomach they just place the ring around it. They made it seem very nice.

The reality was another thing. Patients with bands

didn't fair to well walking into restaurants. The first thing they would look for is the bathroom. Because, well, in case you were feeling sick or you were puking from the food your ordered you have to know where the bathroom is. The healthy food, you just can't eat. You want to try a chicken breast, uh uh, you want to try some produce, uh uh, you want to try some junk food, uh huh, that goes down nice. What the hell!

The thing is, quality of life with band isn't as you picture it. So right now we do a lot of revisions. It's called revisional surgery and you just go from one procedure to another. By the way, I did a revisional band to sleeve surgery on my mom. My mom's story is on our YouTube channel here's the link... www.youtube.com/endobariatric go to playlist and look for "Dr. Alvarez's Mom's Journey"..

Once you have selected your patient do you have a pre-surgery protocol?

I take this decision first. I screen the health histories. Then I give out just the specifics to my coordinator. One patient may have to do a 30-day liquid diet because their BMI is very high. Another patient may have to do a 5-day liquid diet (or 7 days, 10 days, 15 days, depending on specifics). The pre-op diet is based on the intake of liquids. Liquids include protein shakes, meal replacement, creamy soups, yogurts, etcetera, but it's based on fluids. What that does is simply lower the amount of calories you're going to be consuming per day and shrink your liver just before the surgery. Some people say, "Oh doctor you want to make me suffer." No no, it's just for a short period, it's to shrink your liver, then you get surgery and from there on everything will take off.

Can you stretch out your stomach with time?

The take home message is that your stomach will never ever be the size it was before surgery so keep that in mind. You will never ever have that stomach again. But can you stretch it out with time? Yes. Some people freak out. That's six to eight months, maybe a year or two out and they're emailing me. Right after surgery you're at the highest point of inflammation, highest point of restriction. You take one or two bites and you're full. Then you're at a year or two and now you can eat a half of a sandwich. But maybe before surgery you had a complete sandwich, sandwich and a half, potato chips and the soda drink and maybe a muffin for dessert. Always compare that stretch sensation right after surgery to how it was before surgery.

Why are some foods harder to digest?

It's the dryness. Chicken, as with a piece of meat are very dry. It will sit there in your sleeve, you may throw up, but if you eat something with more moistness it will go down easier. Now if you go to extreme dry such as crackers, peanuts, something that doesn't grab moisture in your stomach it will go down easier.

Chapter 45

Coffee, Hormones, Converting A Sleeve, Bougie Size

"When you reduce your body mass you will start to notice you're feeling more energetic, that's those hormones kicking in getting you back on track."

To watch the #AskDrA Show episode that this chapter is based on, follow along at:
www.bit.ly/AskDrA45

How long after surgery can you drink coffee?

I would recommend you stick to decaffeinated coffee the first two weeks after surgery. Here's why, your body needs sleep and pumping caffeine into it may prevent you from getting enough sleep to heal properly. After about 3 weeks you're good to resume regular coffee. So try to wait at least 21 days so your body can adjust to a better sleep pattern.

Which procedure do you suggest for a woman who has never been pregnant?

We get a lot of referrals from OBGYNs about overweight patients who can't get pregnant. They tried all the treatments, just no luck on conceiving. But once sleeved, their fertility goes through the roof. Everything starts to work better. Those hormones kick in and…well, look out.

Everything changed when you were overweight, because If your increase your body mass then you increase your fat tissue which increases estrogen and then that changes everything in your body. You have cycles where you don't ovulate, cycles that you may miss a period, cycles where you just don't know what is happening. But when you bring down your body mass just a bit then everything comes into a perfect cycle.

I have tendency to get keloid scars, how will a sleeve affect me?

Totally independent. Keloid scarring is a build-up of scar tissue around the cut or wound. Maybe it's a bit discolored or thicker. In some cases, women who suffer from PCOS will also experience keloid scarring. The sleeve will help you get into that perfect cycle of your body.

Your PCOS symptoms will go away and your keloid scarring may diminish as well.

Do hormones after surgery tend to spike?

Look at it this way, say there's a sprinkler in the center of the room and it's designed to cover what's in that center only. Now if the center of the room is your body but it's only being covered by some of the sprinkler then we got a problem. That's how hormones work. They are like the sprinkler and they can only cover so much area. When your body is overweight, the hormones just don't cover everything. When you reduce your body mass you will start to notice you're feeling more energetic, that's those hormones kicking in getting you back on track. Less weight means proper hormone coverage.

Can a sleeve be converted into something else?

The cool thing about the sleeve is it can be revised, so if you're thinking about getting a bypass or switch to a gastric bypass that's an option. But you can't go the other way around. Bypass to sleeve can't be done. A sleeve gives you options.

Why do you use a smaller bougie?

Bougie is a French word that means candle. But it's actually the measurement of what we call the calibration to a size of a candle. As you know candles can come in different sizes and thicknesses. But it's that measurement that we use to describe the thickness of the calibration tube that is inserted in your mouth and down your esophagus to your stomach. This tube tells us what pattern or what width to leave that stomach a certain size. The smaller the tube the smaller the capacity, the bigger the tube the bigger the capacity. The smaller the bougie size can keep you in a safety range. You'll be able to eat a spaghetti but vertically.

Chapter 46

Alcohol Sugars, Protein Intake, Resleeving Your Sleeve

"Here in our practice we make sure the patient is eating adequately. We make sure the patient is doing everything in their effort to lose weight."

To watch the #AskDrA Show episode that this chapter is based on, follow along at:
www.bit.ly/AskDrA46

What are your thoughts on sugar alcohols in relation to carbohydrates when choosing certain foods and/or drinks?

Alcohol sugars are sugars that don't have as much impact in the blood regarding the levels of glucose. Your blood glucose doesn't spike up as much with alcohol sugars. If you're counting carbs, you can actually subtract the amount of alcohol sugars from the total amount of carbs, these are your net carbs. It doesn't actually count as net carbs. You have to subtract that because they don't have that much impact on your blood sugar as other carbs do.

I have trouble drinking protein shakes or drinks. How can I get protein in without it?

There are some supplements that are flavorless, odorless that you can mix with some yogurt, that you can mix with some juice or some broth.

Let's say you simply dislike the supplements. Don't worry, your body has enough reserves of protein. You're getting protein even if you're doing just phase one. Let's say you're consuming chicken broth, you're still getting some protein (same goes for vegetable broth and beef broth).

Let's talk about protein intake down the road once you're eating. Drop the supplements. You don't need them. You're still getting enough protein intake. You will not become malnourished because of a lack of protein. Be sure you make wise decisions though. Protein and produce. Focus on protein and produce first, you'll be good. You don't have to be just drinking shakes and supplements all your life. Please understand this. Focus on the food you're in-taking.

Am I able to get a gastric sleeve redone if I haven't lost weight in a year?

We've talked about this before, but I'll share my thoughts once again. The thing is, can it be done, the answer is yes. Can we do it? Yes, we actually

The #AskDrA Book-Vol 2

do it, not that frequently though. We make sure that the patient is a really good candidate for a sleeve the first time, so a redo is not really necessary.

Here in our practice we make sure the patient is eating adequately. We make sure the patient is doing everything in their effort to lose weight. But what if they didn't come to us and their doctor made their stomach big or it was a bad technique or it was a bad sleeve from the get go? Then an endoscopy or a barium swallow would determine the condition the stomach is in. Then we can decide if the patient is a good candidate for resleeving. Don't say you're just stuck. You may only be 10 or 20 pounds away from your goal.

You don't need to resleeve your sleeve. Just make sure you're doing good, eating correctly and making wise decisions.

Chapter 47

Electrolytes, Constipation, How Often Should You Get On The Scale

"I know this is super hard for some to do. Yet it's very important. The best way to measure your progress is your clothes. Clothes don't lie."

To watch the #AskDrA Show episode that this chapter is based on, follow along at: www.bit.ly/AskDrA47

Is my sleeve preventing me from absorbing electrolytes I use to keep me from being dehydrated?

The answer is no. Electrolytes normally get absorbed in the intestine. Remember that the sleeve does not get rerouted into the intestines, so the absorption of electrolytes is at 100%. It does not vary. Put your mind at ease, electrolytes get absorbed 100%. They will not be any malabsorption, and you won't have deficiency of these because of the sleeve itself.

What can be done to prevent constipation as soon as surgery is done?

If you had constipation before surgery, you're more likely to have it afterwards. Now, it's not common that if you didn't have constipation you will develop it afterwards. Normally, if you used to have it, you'll have it. If you didn't, probably you won't have it. Put your mind at ease, it has no direct relationship to the surgery or the sleeve.

Now, right after surgery people who do have constipation, may get constipated. How to avoid it? Patients normally take a soft stool softener. You can take Miralax. You can add a little bit of fiber. You can use Metamucil. You can contact your doctor directly. Of course, my patients have my direct email. You can email me and we can give you few suggestions on how to avoid or treat the constipation, but the point is... don't forget to count your fluid intake. It's very important to stay hydrated. If you're not well hydrated, constipation will follow. Even though you do a stool softener, even if you do fiber, you need the water intake, you need the fluid intake, so actually it can help you with the medication or the stool softener.

How often should I weight myself?

Please don't get on the scale every single day. Let me tell you why. Right after people get the surgery, they're discharged and before they're going home, they want to get on my scale again. I tell them please don't get on the scale, you'll be disappointed. I mean you'll be just in shock, because the scale will move up. Why is this? Because of all the IV fluids that were placed in you during surgery.

IV fluids will take a few days for the body to actually readjust and you'll pee it out and then you'll notice that the scale will start to drop.

The best way is get on the scale every 7 to 10 days. Don't get on the scale sooner than 7 days. Now, I know this is super hard for some to do. Yet it's very important. Best way to measure your progress is your clothes. Clothes don't lie. Your scale will move forward. It'll move down progressively slowly.

Please, please just remember this is a long-term process. You're looking at 10-12 months down the road. Don't think this is going to work the first month and you're going to lose 50 pounds right away. No, no, no, no.

Remember, during this period of time, you will have some stalls and these stalls are normal. Please keep that in mind. They're normal. You don't need to freak out because you hit a stall. You don't need to call 911 because you hit a stall or plateau. Remember that these stalls are needed for your body. Your body is readjusting. I mean your body needs to readjust, and these adjustments occur frequently and your body will continue advancing.

I have some patients that will just weigh themselves on my scale every time they visit. "I don't get on any other scale. I just use yours doctor," which is great. They see the progress with their clothes, they start to feel different and everything, and they use one scale every 2 or 3 months once they come to visit us. The take-home message is don't get obsessed by using the scale.

Chapter 48

Blood Clots, Reducing Diabetes Medications, Eating Meat

"Take your time eating and remind yourself that you need to chew very well."

To watch the #AskDrA Show episode that this chapter is based on, follow along at: www.bit.ly/AskDrA48

Is it true that flying after surgery can cause blood clots?

The short answer is no. If everyone who ever had surgery experienced blood clots when flying, nobody would fly anymore. Here's the slightly longer answer...blood clots can form or are more associated with forming on flights longer than 4 hours. It's not the plane that's the problem...it's the length of time sitting in the same position without moving around. What you can do to help prevent clotting is move about. Get up, stretch and walk. Of course, you should wait until you hear the captain say it's okay. Walking the aisles, standing, stretching and moving about helps. And wearing compression socks or stockings is also something we recommend which will help prevent clotting.

Can we reduce insulin and other diabetes meds during pre-operation diet?

If you're on 1, 2 or several medications for diabetes, it is important for you to know or let your doctor know that you are going to do a pre-op diet to get you in shape for surgery. It is important for you to get your primary health physician or internist on board prior to starting your pre-op diet. After surgery you will be consuming less calories per day and will be needing to adjust your medications.

I have trouble eating meat. Any advice?

Eating drier food like chicken breast, a rib eye or a chunk of meat is difficult the first 6 months. Remember to take an antacid and make sure the meat you are eating is cut into smaller pieces. Take your time and remind yourself that you need to chew very well.

Chapter 49

Feeling Lightheaded, Bruising, Using An App To Count Calories

"Make sure you're taking your supplements, that you're eating correctly, not skipping meals, and you'll be just fine."

To watch the #AskDrA Show episode that this chapter is based on, follow along at: www.bit.ly/AskDrA49

I have been feeling really light-headed and have an excessive amount of bruises popping up. Is it normal after 6-months post-operation?

Feeling light-headed, yes, normal. Having a lot of bruising, combined with lightheadedness then it's a red flag. Make sure, you are not skipping meals, you're eating the correct amount of calories and you're taking your vitamins. It's very important you're taking your vitamins and supplements, and not skipping them.

Bruising is a good sign that you're lacking vitamin K. Vitamin K is important. If you're not taking your supplements, and you're missing out on vitamin K, that's a problem. Make sure you're taking your supplements, that you're eating correctly, not skipping meals, and you'll be just fine.

Is it okay to use an appetite suppressant during the pre-operation diet?

Well, let me tell you the pre-op diet is doable. We don't give you anything that's impossible to do. Normally, we have you cut down on calories, and increase your fluid intake. You can use appetite suppressants if you truly need to, but why? You really need to do this using them. But if you must use them, then it's okay.

But FYI...the vast majority of patients are able to do this without any prescription medications, and it's a doable diet.

Any recommendations for protein, carb, and calorie tracking apps?

Yes. My Fitness Pal, that's my favorite one, available for Android. It's also available for Blackberry, but then again, who uses Blackberry nowadays? And, you can also download for Apple devices. I use it every single day. I track calories. I track carbs. If you go to the premium version, tracks the amount carbs, protein and the fat you intake. You also get the interaction with certain devices like Garmin.

Also, most important thing, it also creates this awareness of where calories may be hidden and what you might be able to eat in more quantity.

Chapter 50

Creams, Throat Sensation, Buffalo Hump

"When you do your part your sleeve will do its part, and you'll get the best possible outcome."

To watch the #AskDrA Show episode that this chapter is based on, follow along at: www.bit.ly/AskDrA50

When is it okay to start using products like skin firming lotions and creams after the surgery?

Let's talk about keeping your skin hydrated…that's the best thing you can do to get positive results down the road. To avoid the loose skin or maybe have less loose skin you need to keep your skin hydrated. Use a hydration lotion in the morning and in the evening. It may be kind of a hassle, but if you use it you will get the best outcomes.

I feel like something is stuck in my throat. I'm two weeks post operation. What could it be?

Right after surgery, you may have that sensation that something is stuck. That sensation is actually that you ate too much. Or you swallowed too much. Or you gulped water down very quickly. Or you're at the liquid phase and you're taking it too fast. The liquid or food gets stuck in your esophagus which may cause a spasm, causing that sensation that something is really stuck. It isn't. My best suggestion is take it slow, make sure you're following your diet or your diet phase. If you're already eating, be sure to eat very slow, chew very well, and you'll avoid the sensation.

Is it possible that our buffalo hump neck fat will go away or shrink down?

Although this may sound like a weird question, some patients do want to know how to get rid of it. Typically, when I gain weight, I gain it in my thighs or my back, but some of you may experience that little hump. That lump or hump may go away once you start losing weight. Maybe it's the way you gain fat in your body, but once you lose this fat it may go away. I have seen plastic surgeons actually just go attack that area. But honestly for simplicity sake, just let your sleeve do its job. When you do your part your sleeve will do its part, and you'll get the best possible outcome. Normally, that hump will go away. I've seen it go away on many patients. Yet, as with everything in life, results will vary from person to person. If you have a little hump that just doesn't go away a little liposuction in that area and it's gone.

Chapter 51

Weight Stalls, Daily Fluid Intake, Passports To Mexico

"If you're experiencing very, very hot weather you need to increase the amount of water daily. Keep track."

To watch the #AskDrA Show episode that this chapter is based on, follow along at: www.bit.ly/AskDrA51

At what point should I be concerned that I'm at a stall in my weight loss?

Let's talk about weight stalls. I've said it once...I'll say it again. Weight stalls are normal. Weight stalls are needed. Plateaus are needed for your body to adjust. Please understand that your body is going through a lot of stress. Through a lot of changes. Your body needs to adapt. Your body needs to put a stall and say, "Wait a minute. I need to readjust certain functions." Like, hormones. Like the amount of fluid in your body. Like the amount of blood in your body. Your cardiopulmonary functions. All those things change. Why? Well, let's say you start out before sleeve surgery at 300lbs or more. And now after surgery, you're 150 pounds or lighter. That's an incredible difference on your body. Those stalls are needed to readjust to the changes.

When should I worry if I hit a stall? Well, the stalls can last a week. They can last 2 weeks. They can last 5 weeks, 6 weeks and even 7 weeks. Those stalls could last a few months. What you need to do is keep track of your progress. And, keep focused. If you're still exercising and burning some calories, you're doing fine. Make sure you get enough fluids.

All you have to do is just wait and the weight stall will go away. You'll break it. You'll continue losing weight and continue losing size. Please just keep in mind that you need to keep focused while you're hitting the stall.

How much fluid should I intake on average each day to minimize chances of dehydration?

How much fluid do you need? You need 64 ounces. Plain and simple, all right? But, it's going to be practically impossible for you to drink 64 ounces right after surgery. Specially, the first few days. Why? Because this sleeve is just barely crafted. It's still swollen in there. You'll be able to sip, wait, sip, wait. You'll be able to do that but it's very difficult to get to the 64 ounces right away. As the days go by, (maybe day 4 or day 5), it gets much easier, and you'll be able to get enough fluids.

People with sleeves have a difficult time with water. It's much harder to get that water down than any other regular fluid, like tea for example.

Mixing water with Gatorade or Crystal light will change the water's osmolarity, and make that water easier to go down. If you have initially some trouble with plain water, switch or add something to that water and it changes the whole deal. You need to hit 64 ounces.

If you're experiencing very, very hot weather you need to increase the amount of water daily. Keep track.

I was wondering if I would need a passport to come for surgery.

Back in the old days, you didn't need a passport to come to Mexico for a surgery because it was ground transportation. Nowadays, you don't need a passport to come into Mexico but you do need a passport to get back into the United States. So the correct answer is yes, you do need it. It's a simple process. You will need it sooner or later. Might as well just get the passport. You can use it in the future for traveling.

Chapter 52

Gallstones, Thrill Rides & Eating Lettuce

"Check with your surgeon and their programs. Follow their guidelines and you shouldn't have any problems."

To watch the #AskDrA Show episode that this chapter is based on, follow along at:
www.bit.ly/AskDrA52

Why do so many weight loss surgery patients end up with gallstone problems?

Some people worry a little too much about developing gallstones and maybe holding back on having weight loss surgery because of the fear of "what if". Let's talk a little bit about what procedures cause gallstones or may make you prone to develop gallstones easier.

Malabsorption procedures that cause you to lose really rapid weight like gastric bypass and duodenal switch. Not so much with the gastric sleeve which is a more restrictive procedure. I tell patients, "Look at it this way. If you were prone to have gallstones at any point in your life, the weight loss will actually precipitate the development of gallstones sooner. You're going to have them anyway."

Don't worry about if you develop gallstones down the road. Gallbladder surgeries are done every single day. It's a very safe procedure. Don't let it hold you back on having weight loss surgery, having a better quality of life. If you're thinking that postponing the sleeve surgery because you might have gallstones down the road. Don't worry about it if you were going to have them you're going to get them anyway with or without weight loss surgery.

When can I get on thrill rides?

Thrill rides are completely safe for the sleeve 30 days after surgery. You may get on thrill rides that are not too intense maybe at 21 days, but my recommendation is wait at least 30 days.

When it is safe to add the lettuce salad options?

I would make sure you check with your surgeon and his programs. In our program it's 21 days, so after 21 days your stomach is healed. You can start adding some soft food including some salad, some lettuce. I don't want to interfere with your surgeon's program. Make sure you're following his or her guidelines and you won't have any issues.

Glossary of Terms

Acid Blocker – are a class of medications that reduce or block stomach acids from forming

Acid Reflux – is a chronic condition caused by stomach acid coming up into the esophagus

Alcohol Sugar – is a carbohydrate that has fewer calories than regular sugar and less effect on blood glucose levels.

Antacids – a substance which neutralizes stomach acids

BMI – short for "body mass index"

Bougie – a thin flexible surgical instrument used for exploring or dilating a passage of the body

Buffalo Hump – an excess deposit of fat localized on the back of the neck resembling a hump on a buffalo.

Carbs – short for "carbohydrates"

Creatine – a supplement used for muscle improvement.

Duodenal Switch – a weight loss surgery procedure which removes a portion of the stomach and reroutes a lengthy portion of the small intestines.

Electrolytes – a substance that produces an electrically charged solution when dissolved in water

Endoscopy - a nonsurgical procedure used to examine a person's digestive tract using an endoscope

Fluid Intake – the amount of fluid consumed daily

Glossary of Terms continued...

Gastric Band - is a silicone device placed around the upper section of the stomach, creating a small pouch above the band and thereby restricting the amount of food that can be comfortably eaten

Gastric Bypass - refers to a surgical procedure in which the stomach is divided into a small upper pouch and a much larger lower "remnant" pouch and then the small intestine is rearranged to connect to both.

Gastric Sleeve - is a surgical weight loss procedure in which the stomach is reduced to about 25% of its original size, by surgical removal of a large portion of the stomach along the greater curvature.

Health System – an organization devoted to health care solutions.

Incision - a surgical cut made in skin or flesh.

Invasive - involving entry into the living body (as by incision or by insertion of an instrument)

Intestines - are a long, continuous tube running from the stomach to the anus.

IV Fluids – are liquids, medications or blood used intravenously.

Liquid Phase – anything that has the consistency of what can easily be strained through a straw

Malabsorption - is a state arising from abnormality in absorption of food nutrients across the GI tract.

Malnutrition - is a condition that results from eating a diet in which nutrients are not enough which then causes health problems.

Glossary of Terms continued...

Medical Tourism – is the traveling to another country to obtain medical treatment

Metabolism - is a term that is used to describe all chemical reactions involved in maintaining the living state of the cells and the organism.

NSAIDS – short for "Nonsteroidal anti-inflammatory drugs" such as aspirin, ibuprofen, naproxen

Nausea – the discomfort that you feel before vomiting

OBGYN – short for "Obstetrics & Gynecology."

PCP - short for "primary care physician"

PCOS – short for Polycystic Ovary Syndrome

Potassium – a natural chemical compound that helps with gastrointestinal motility, metabolism and electrolyte balance.

Restrictions – help identify a patient's limitations and capabilities.

Revisional Surgery – is a surgical procedure done to revise a past treatment

Soft Food Phase – food that has the consistency of applesauce

Splenda – a sucralose-based artificial sweetener

VSG – short for "vertical sleeve gastrectomy"

Weight Stall – is a temporary adjustment when after weight loss surgery your body stalls to lose weight.

About The Authors

Dr. Guillermo Alvarez, a premier bariatric surgeon located in Piedras Negras, Coahuila, Mexico who is passionate about helping people fulfill their lifelong desire of attaining better health and a more fulfilling lifestyle. Dr. Alvarez has helped over 10,000 patients gain a new lease on life with the help of the gastric sleeve surgery.

Dr. Alvarez dedicates his practice to helping his patients achieve dramatic weight loss that leads to a healthier, longer and more prosperous life. Following weight loss surgery, many of Dr. Alvarez's patients are soon able to enjoy the benefits and joys of life that they previously could not while suffering from obesity. An improved love life, a more active lifestyle and the ability to enjoy quality time with friends and family are just some of the few positive changes that you will experience after weight loss surgery.

Rob Anspach, an author, speaker and business strategist located in Lancaster County, Pennsylvania, USA who is passionate about changing lives. Mr. Anspach serves as the Coordinator for The Endobariatric Foundation, and the Founder of Anspach Media.

Mr. Anspach is also the author of "Social Media Debunked", "Share: 27 Ways To Boost Your Social Media Experience, Build Trust and Attract Followers", "Optimize This: How Two Carpet Cleaners Consistently Beat Web Designers On The Search Engines" and "Lessons From The Dojo: 101 Ways To Improve Your Life, Business and Relationships".

Endobariatric

Dr. Alvarez's bariatric surgery Mexico facility is updated frequently to stay ahead of the normal standards used in the USA. The operating room is equipped with an emergency power plant that guarantees continuous electrical supply in case of an emergency such as an uncommon blackout. The hospital has a wide variety of diagnostic equipment that is found in large hospitals in the States, such as an MRI, Helicoidal CT Scan, Doppler Sonogram, etc.

This hospital has the top intensive care unit in this region with a staff of doctors and nurses that specialize in any trauma or emergency to support our patients in any case needed. You can feel safe in knowing that the staff of this facility is more than capable in handling your needs as a patient. The hospital is considered a "Specialized" hospital to handle the most difficult individual cases that are present.

The hospital includes 35 private rooms for patients and guest. Each room has telephone, TV, cable and a place for your guests to sleep. There are 4 suites available that also have a sofa and recliner.

The nursing staff is very professional and well trained for your care as a bariatric patient. There are 3 shifts (as opposed to the states - 2 shifts). We feel that is important that our entire team is fresh and alert to keep a 24-hour monitoring protocol. This entire staff is more than capable in handling all of your post-op care.

This hospital is a wonderful place for our bariatric patients to experience a safe and calm atmosphere and an excellent outcome during your recovery period. If you are considering this surgery for yourself or a family member, feel free to contact us any time. This is an option that will ensure you the best care from an excellent team of surgeons, nurses and top-notch hospital. We will be happy to have one of our coordinators assist you with more information and pricing.

1(866)697-5338 www.Endobariatric.com

Endo-Foundation

The Endobariatric Foundation is dedicated to helping those who truly desire to have the gastric sleeve procedure done, but might not have all the funds available to do so.

The ultimate goal of the foundation is to help those who are struggling financially avoid making the mistake of choosing a cheap gastric sleeve surgeon because they didn't have enough money.

"Money should never be that speed bump that slows you down and prevents you from improving your life".

So here's what we are doing to insure the success of the Foundation and make sure there are resources available when patients apply. We are setting aside a portion of every bill from every paying client and using it to fund this very worthwhile endeavor. This will be part of the Endobariatric legacy and will mean so much to so many.

To apply for a Foundation grant to help with your gastric sleeve surgery visit **www.Endofoundation.com** today.

Become a Sponsor!

If you like to help people as much as we do, we invite you to become a sponsor. It can be a simple one-time gift of $25 or you can sponsor every month for whatever amount you deem life changing.

Mail your sponsorship monies to:

Endobariatric, SC
P.O. Box 6529 Eagle Pass TX 78853

Endo-Spa

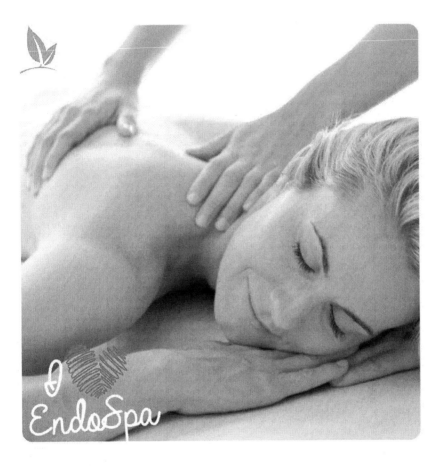

With relaxing surroundings, innovative treatments and a talented staff, EndoSpa nurtures your body, invigorates your senses and relaxes your mind. EndoSpa offers a wide array of spa treatments for men and women.

Massage – Facials – Laser Treatment

Hair Removal – Acoustic Wave Therapy

www.EndoSpa.mx

Endo-Store

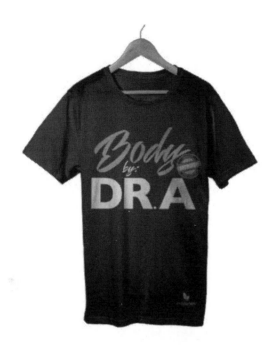

- Shirts
- Hats
- Bags
- Bottles
- Pillows
- Books
And more!

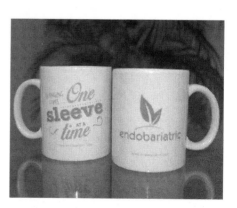

www.EndoStoreOnline.com

The Book That Started The Series

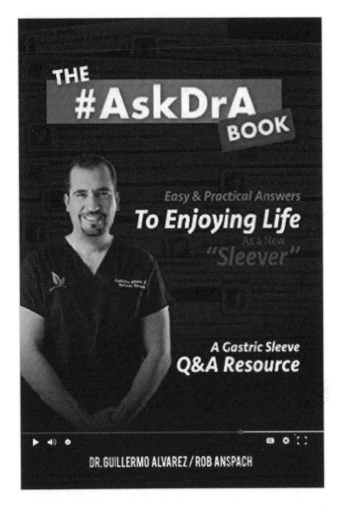

Dr. Guillermo Alvarez / Rob Anspach

Available on Amazon

& EndoStoreOnline.com

Other Books By The Authors

Dr. Guillermo Alvarez

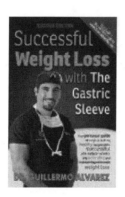 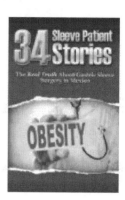

Rob Anspach

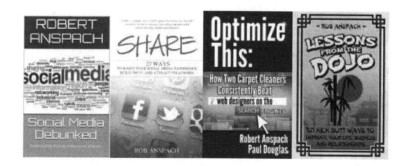

Available on Amazon

Be A Fan!

Follow Dr. Alvarez
on these Social Networks.

Facebook - www.facebook.com/endobariatric

Google+ - https://plus.google.com/+Endobariatric

Twitter - www.twitter.com/endobariatric

Pinterest - www.pinterest.com/endobariatric

Instagram - www.instagram.com/endobariatric

LinkedIn - www.linkedin.com/in/endobariatric

YouTube - www.youtube.com/endobariatric

Snapchat - www.snapchat.com/add/gmoalvarez

If you have a question and would like to get it answered...post it to Facebook, Twitter, Instagram or YouTube with the hashtag #AskDrA

Or send your question via Snapchat.

We might even answer it on our weekly show or in the next book.

Share This Book!

I mean it!

Tell your friends all about this book.

Share where you bought it.

Share it at lunch!

Share it at the gym!

Share it on the beach!

Share it on social media.

Share it using this hashtag...

TheAskDrABook2

Made in the USA
Columbia, SC
21 June 2019